OUTSPOKEN Nursing

RN success in today's economy

OUTSPOKEN Nursing

RN success in today's economy

Ashley T. Parham, MSN, RN, CNE

ISBN-13: 978-0-578-44993-7

Dedication

This book is dedicated to my grandmother, Susan Morris, whose health status has been deteriorating due to dementia. While she has experienced some slight improvements, she is not the same – not as I remember her to be. I love her to pieces, and when she overcame Stage IV breast cancer while I was in nursing school, I just knew she would be around "forever". Unfortunately, her body is changing. I simply pray for the healthcare providers and my family involved in her care. I love nursing and I believe in healthcare, so grandma, this is for you!

I'm thankful for my husband and two girls who have allowed me to love what I do in a way that is not always comfortable for them. I absolutely love nursing – and all its associated baggage! I am also thankful for their continuous support for every new and unique endeavor I undertake. My family is always there even nursing sometimes seems like a lonely place.

This is also dedicated to any nursing colleagues I have cared for patients with or taught nursing students with that have expressed a genuine concern about healthcare and/or nursing education. I have had the opportunity to work with and work for some DYNAMIC healthcare leaders – that just so happen to be nurses. Even more, I have worked with spectacular nursing students that have provided me deeper insight into the need for transparency at all levels of healthcare.

Table of Contents

Preface

I want to begin by first saying that I genuinely respect all obstetric (OB) healthcare professionals. I would also like to add that I am not at all a fan of obstetric ANYTHING. I have felt this way since I was in nursing school, and after having my first child, my distasteful feelings for OB only increased. While I had a spectacular team of healthcare professionals working with me during the delivering of my first child, the experience was very traumatic. I remember feeling like I knew everything there was to know about breathing during contractions, epidurals, how to push a baby out, and how nice the labor and delivery room was going to be – as compared to the rest of the hospital. What I did not know was how painful pushing a baby out was going to be.

I know...you're probably thinking "Seriously? Are you for real? Of course, it's painful!" Honestly, I was so wrapped up in the perfect idea of "delivering" a beautiful baby and being able to swaddle her, change her diaper correctly, have her nursery all set, and have all my breastfeeding plans together. I didn't think about much else. All the videos, books, and even the baby classes talk about pushing through the pain, but they don't quite describe the pain as "horror". For me, the "pain" would have been better termed as "horror".

My name is Ashley and the horror went like this:

1) Perfect contractions with absolutely no pain all the way to 8 cm dilation
2) So of course, I did not need an epidural
3) Immediately and out of nowhere, my pain went from 0/10 (none) to 8/10 (pretty bad)
4) "Give me the epidural now!"
5) The anesthesiologist was probably very used to patients like me, but I was not used to myself. How can I sit still on the side of a bed to get an epidural when I am already in so much horrific pain? Oh, and by the way, it felt like I was sitting on a baby!
6) While the epidural may have been working, I had already morphed into "a crazy" by that point, so no additional OB medication was going to change my "crazy" – I couldn't focus. I literally went from being "Ashley" to being ... "CRASHLEY". It was bad.
7) Right before delivery (during shift change), my spectacular physicians were at the foot of the bed - very SAFELY giving report to one another to change shifts. Watching this happen – physicians talking instead of getting my baby out – made me angry and made me feel like I was in even more pain.
8) Finally, the horrific pain was over, and my beautiful daughter came into the world.
9) My husband then proceeded to say, "So I guess we won't be having any more kids for a while?"

I felt so unprepared for the type of pain that ensued and I don't like being caught off guard. I may have even told my family that they should have told me about the pain! Everyone says, "You forget all about the pain once you see your baby's face". Yeah, that didn't quite happen with me. I definitely remembered the pain very vividly until about my daughter's first birthday. Needless to say, I read nothing about diaper changing and swaddling when it came to the next child. I went into the Labor and Delivery (L&D) room like I was preparing to play in the Olympics – game face on and ready.

So what does my birthing experience have to do with this book? I believe success and improvement comes through understanding and transparency. While I would have liked to receive this type of transparency prior to my delivery, I realize I should have owned some responsibility for being transparent with myself. Success occurs when we are clear about what actually happens vs. what should happen. Only then can we see areas for growth and we are able to see ourselves in that growing process. Becoming a nurse and developing in the nursing field requires an immense amount of growth as an individual. While developing as a nurse, we must also recognize that the healthcare field is also growing and changing at an even faster rate. Therefore, it is imperative that we are aware of our contextual influences when trying to grow as an individual.

My birthing experience is not quite the experience I had in my nursing career; however, it is relatively similar. Unfortunately, nursing school cannot prepare you for everything; as a bulk of the preparation must focus on patient care and medical knowledge application. Had I not been blessed to have so many beautiful nurses in my life to help me and provide guidance, wisdom, and their own personal stories, I would have struggled more with some of the realities that come with trying to develop as a new nurse in a dynamic career field and healthcare environment.

My intent for this book is not to steer anyone away from nursing, but to be very transparent – as much as I possibly can – to be sure that people are aware of the career they are going into. This way they can be more successful by being mentally prepared, rather than feeling beat up by an imperfect healthcare system because they were repetitively caught off guard. Working in healthcare can be great, but it's not always pretty. I hope that through transparency and appropriate preparation, you will feel capable of recognizing and handling the many challenges, while recognizing positive gains for self-fulfillment and continually moving in the direction of improving healthcare.

Disclosure

The opinions in this book are solely my own and do not represent any of my current or former employers, colleagues or any other large or small nursing or healthcare organizations. My opinions in this book do not represent nursing as a profession, healthcare as a whole, or any organizations I am affiliated with. I received no form of payment for citing any of the articles in this book. The articles mentioned were chosen due to their relation to the content discussed in the chapter and I personally view them as valuable articles for reading. Recommendations, opinions, and statements made in this book do not guarantee success in any career path; they are only recommendations that might be helpful, but are not absolutes.

First things first – Defining “success”

What does “success” look like?

You are the only person who can define what success looks like to you. Over time, you will learn that your definition of success will change as you grow, develop, learn more about the world, learn more about yourself, and as the context of the world around you continues to change. Think about what “success” means to you. After you have finished reading this book, be sure to contemplate on this regularly as life changes – and it will change frequently.

Seriously.

STOP.

Take about 3-5 minutes (or more) to think about what success in life looks like or might look like to you.

Chapter 1: Routes to becoming a Registered Nurse

ADN, BSN, MSN...turn left, turn right, look up, look down; they all lead you to becoming an RN

There are many routes to becoming a registered nurse (RN). Each route has its own potential advantages and potential disadvantages. My description of these advantages and disadvantages are purely subjective, and do not always apply. Although, before even beginning to look at the different routes to becoming an RN, you must know that prior to taking either of these routes, you need to first take prerequisite courses. These are courses that are required prior to applying for nursing school. They often provide you with a base of knowledge about the human body, basic sciences, etc. Prerequisite courses for all nursing schools (even within the same state) are NOT always the same, so be sure to obtain the exact required prerequisite course list in order to qualify for admission into a particular nursing program.

Now, do not confuse degree graduation requirements with prerequisites. *What are you talking about Ashley?* I "mean" that some people like to rush and get into nursing school and attempt to take degree required courses, such as World History II, while they are fulltime nursing students. Depending on the type of nursing program you will be in, taking those types of additional courses may make nursing school even more challenging. If provided the opportunity, attempt to take your degree required courses – as much as possible – prior to beginning nursing school. Information regarding what basic courses are required to obtain an associate, bachelor's, or master's degree are usually found within the school's registrar or student services department. Most often, you can obtain a course guide from the school of nursing prior to entering the nursing program so you can begin planning how you can fulfill your graduation requirements.

Again, each nursing program may have different prerequisites, so be sure to look at the nursing programs you are interested in and do not assume all schools have the same requirements. READ, READ, READ. Now let's look at some different types of nursing programs.

ADN = Associates Degree in Nursing
BSN = Bachelor of Science in Nursing
MSN = Master of Science in Nursing

Associate Degree Programs

- ADN programs are often offered at community colleges

Perceived ADVANTAGES	Perceived DISADVANTAGES
1. Cost savings: Community colleges or other schools that offer ADN programs often charge less per credit hour – compared to larger schools and/or BSN programs.	1. All nursing courses may not transfer to a BSN program; you MUST check. a. *Resulting in potentially more costs overall – in comparison to just attending a BSN program.*
2. Some courses at the ADN level may transfer to a BSN program.	2. Some facilities will not hire ADN nurses (they may require at least a BSN)
3. You may get paid the same as a BSN and/or entry-level MSN in some facilities in in some cities.	

Bachelor's Degree Programs

- BSN programs are often offered at 4-year colleges and/or universities

Perceived ADVANTAGES	Perceived DISADVANTAGES
1. Many facilities would prefer the BSN student over the ADN student comparably	1. Often costlier per credit hour than ADN programs

Bachelor-to-Master's Degree Programs

- BSN to MSN programs are offered at 4-year colleges and/or universities

Perceived ADVANTAGES	Perceived DISADVANTAGES
1. These types of programs often lead you to becoming an advanced practice nurse.	1. You have limited experience as a staff RN prior to becoming a leader of healthcare teams. This does not always present problems for everyone – it depends on your personality and/or environment.

Perceived ADVANTAGES	Perceived DISADVANTAGES
2. There is usually no expectation for you to have experience as an RN prior to beginning the MSN program.	2. There will be organizations/institutions that value experience over education. a. *Some institutions may prefer hiring someone with previous staff nurse experience and/or previous advanced practice nursing experience.*
3. You will be able to move from having no nursing degree to obtaining your advanced practice nursing degree in a shorter time frame.	

Direct-Entry Master's Degree Programs

- These MSN programs are offered at 4-year colleges and/or universities with graduate nursing programs

Perceived ADVANTAGES	Perceived DISADVANTAGES
1. Oftentimes, in order to qualify for these programs, you must first have a bachelor's degree in another field. This type of program is nice because you can enter the nursing field without having to spend time and money obtaining another bachelor's degree first. You can completely skip the BSN.	1. Costlier than many other programs, as the student will be paying graduate rates per credit hour.
2. Should you decide to go further after this degree and become an NP, you will have already taken some graduate level core courses.	2. You will usually still graduate with an entry level nursing degree and will not be considered an advanced practice nurse (APRN).
3. You will qualify for many types of positions that require a master's degree. Even more, you will qualify for those that require a master's	3. Depending on the facility or city you work in, you may be paid the same amount as a new graduate from an ADN program. This means

Perceived ADVANTAGES	Perceived DISADVANTAGES
degree "nursing". If this degree is not an Advanced Practice degree, you may still qualify for some jobs because of the "MSN" alone.	that every facility does not reward you for your higher degree when you have the same job title – staff RN.

<u>Additional Resource:</u> A great site to gather additional information is the American Nurses Association[1] website. This site discusses how to become a nurse and provides more information about the nursing field.

References

American Nurses Association. *How to become a nurse*. Retrieved on January 16, 2019 from https://www.nursingworld.org/practice-policy/workforce/what-is-nursing/how-to-become-a-nurse/

Chapter 2: How will you pay for school?!?!

Money, Money, Money…MONEY!

Student loans

Student loans or any loans are never the best option for paying for anything, however, for many, this is the only way school may ever be an option. The main thing to always be sure of is the type of loan that's being obtained, the lenders, and the interest rates. The other key point about student loans… NEVER take out more than you need. While you may be broke (having limited funds) during nursing school and still want to "enjoy college life", enjoy it on your own money. Should you choose to take out more loans than you need, you will be charged interest on that money and will probably regret it later in life.

Think about it this way…you can eventually make a salary of about $100,000, and because of student loan decisions made in college, it can feel like you are making $60,000. Aside from the gap in what you could make verses what you will actually feel from day-to-day (100,000 vs 60,000), you will more than likely be working "hard" for the $100,000 – again, only feeling like about $60,000 is hitting your pocket. Consider the other things you would like to do in life after nursing school, such as starting a family, getting married, traveling, etc. Believe me, I know this feeling. My decision to get a student loan was not an easy one, but an obligation to pay my tuition. Just less than 1.5 years ago – while married with two kids – I was living in a two-bedroom apartment and am still trying to pay off my loans. It can feel rough sometimes...and cramped. I refused to live outside my means and place my family at risk in doing so. I also knew I needed an MSN in order to be happy doing what I love the way I wanted to do it.

Additional Resource: These articles/news reports discuss the impact of student loans a bit further.

- ✓ *When does my future begin? Student debt and intragenerational mobility.*
- ✓ *Soaring student loan debt poses risk to nation's future economic growth.*

Scholarships

Scholarships are always one of the best options (usually), but they are not always available. If you haven't been searching up, down, left and right for scholarships, start now. You would be surprised the type of scholarships that you may qualify for. There are many out there with lots of money to spread around. Start looking early! As a matter of fact, it's never too early (and never too late). If you are in high school and begin looking, you will have time to work on projects that current scholarships may require whenever you are ready to apply.

Some scholarships require you to choose a particular path in nursing. If you begin looking early, you may find that a certain path suits your interests.

When looking for scholarships, think about every aspect of your life. What is unique about you and how will that help our country or our world? Thinking in such a manner can help you find certain scholarships that are unique to you – and potentially provide you with less competition. Examples of your unique walk of life could include: being Hispanic, being a musician, being African American, being an American Red Cross volunteer, volunteering at a VA hospital, interest in veterans, being a military dependent, being a cancer survivor, etc.

Grants

Grants, much like scholarships, are often described as "free money". This is because there is usually no expectation for the grant funding to be repaid. Grants are often need-based. If you qualify, grants can be one of the best financial options for paying for school. Certain instances may call for portions or all of the grant funds to be repaid. This could be due to lack of completion of an academic program or lack of completion of the agreed upon requirements.

Funds or financial support from your current employer

Some employers provide funding for employees to go back to school. Great employers realize that their organization is as strong as their weakest employees. Many times, the employee receiving these types of educational funds is required to make some type of commitment to their company. Depending on the company policy, this commitment can be served while you are in school or may only be served after you have completed the degree. For some, this can be a great opportunity to have school paid for, while others may view this as a "commitment trap". Everyone rightfully has their own opinion, as everyone has different plans for the direction of their lives.

How will your payment method affect you and your lifestyle after graduation?

This is the most important aspect of choosing your financial payment method. Consider your future plans and think about how your payment method will affect your lifestyle during and after nursing school. Be sure to read every detail of everything you sign and fully understand any associated obligation that comes with your signature!

References

Elliot, W., Rauscher, E. (2018). When does my future begin? Student debt and intragenerational mobility. *Sociology Mind,* 8, 175-201. doi: 10.4236/sm.2018.82015

Federal Student Aid. (2019). Grants and scholarships. Retrieved from https://studentaid.ed.gov/sa/types/grants-scholarships

Puzzanghera, J. (2015, September 05). Soaring student loan debt poses risk to nation's future economic growth. *Los Angeles Times*. Retrieved from http://www.latimes.com/business/la-fi-student-debt-20150906-story.html

Chapter 3: What to expect from nursing school

Nursing school is hard! BOOM! That's what you should expect.

It's Hard

Many people – even health professionals – have a very misguided idea of what nurses do. To be quite honest, I had no idea about what nurses did until I began nursing school. Yes, I am one of those that were able to get through school (high school and college) with comfort and ease and it never dawned on me that I would have to "get a job" at some point in life. Initially, I was preparing to go to medical school and had a change of heart. While my "heart and mind" were still processing my "life plan", I knew I had to decide quickly. Sitting at my mother's house while trying to plan my life was not an option. So, I figured I would "try" ...nursing. I didn't really know what it was all about. I literally slipped up into a direct-entry master's degree program and quickly learned to love "the nurse" and its many "personalities".

As I'm writing this, I am still trying to find a way to explain what it is that we do without using such "profound" language, so that the nursing roles and responsibilities do not sound so grandiose. The reality of this job is just this – in layman's terms:

<u>My LONG definition of a Registered Nurse</u>

A registered nurse is someone who uses scientific knowledge and critical thinking to recognize changes in a patient's status, determines potential contributing factors to those status changes, promotes optimal healthy living to patients that may or may not want to change their lifestyle in ways that will be heard and received by the patient, educates patients and families about how to care for themselves using charts, pictures, equipment, teach back methods, etc., educates patients on how to troubleshoot equipment, educates patients about medications and diets, administers medications of many types, multitasks throughout the entire day, makes quick decisions and speaks up appropriately in times of chaos or emergencies, stays abreast with new healthcare information (evidence-based practice – EBP), incorporates that new information in the way they care for patients, sits with patients, families, friends, children, and parents during times of uncertainty, sadness, and joy, sticks you with a needle one minute, and gives you a hug the next, empowers their patients and families to ask questions and take the reins on their own healthcare, helps give patients bed baths or showers and then continues to respect the patient as if there body were never exposed to anyone, cries at night in bed after work because they wish they could have taken away all the patient's pain, gets emotionally unstable when they hear of great news about a patient they have cared for, calls everyone on the team to be sure their patient gets every possible appropriate resource before sending the patient out the door, makes/changes beds to be sure patients don't feel like they are living in a prison, learns from their patients every day, pays attention to every single detail all the time – even outside of the hospital – because they have learned to be in constant "assessment" mode, and pushes through the fatigue of yesterday's work. Lastly, a RN is someone who genuinely believes in the idea of a healthier world for every individual – no matter ethnicity, background or economic status.

And this is not an Advanced Practiced RN – this is the description of a staff nurse. I'm pretty sure I'm leaving out many details to the RN's roles and responsibilities as well.

My short definition of a Register Nurse

A registered nurse is someone who does everything under the sun to help patients – often with limited resources and/or time. So, when you hear people say, "Nursing school is/was hard." Well, it should be. Everything that was just described as my "long definition for a RN" is just how an RN may care for 1 patient at the surface level. Mind you, in a day's work, an RN may care for about 4-5 patients at a time... Again, I'm not even talking about nurse practitioners or nurse anesthetists; I'm only referring to staff nurses (staff RNs).

If you were a patient and your nurse told you his/her nursing school was "easy peasy" .... how would that make you feel as a patient?

Additional Resource: The article, "Healthcare Transformation and the Changing Roles for Nursing" (2017), shows just how intertwined nurses are in healthcare. We are or should be in the center of literally everything – every decision, every change, every communication effort, etc. If you are not yet a nurse, or not in the healthcare field and are struggling to read this article with understanding, attempt it, and then feel free to come back to these.

References

Salmond, S., Echevarria, M. (2017). Healthcare Transformation and Changing Roles for Nursing. *Orthopedic nursing*. 36(1), 12-25. Doi: 10.1097/NOR.0000000000000308

Chapter 4: Surviving nursing school

Understanding what it looks like. Again, nursing school is not easy.

Didactic

Just in case you haven't heard the term "didactic". Didactic refers to the classroom learning environment (lecture in the classroom or online, classroom group activities, etc.). Didactics are one component of some of your nursing courses. These are the beginning phases of learning. In the classroom, you should expect to review and learn "textbook" information and learn how to critically think about information.

Medical Simulation
What is this and is it valuable?

Many nursing schools are leading the way in medical simulation. Medical simulation provides all learners, to include nursing students, the opportunity to care for simulated patients in a safe environment. Yes, this is the place where you get to practice what you have learned on pretend patients – manikins, peers, etc. This is sometimes done by practicing a procedural skill only, practicing verbal communication, or even by putting multiple concepts and skills together in one simulated patient scenario. Simulation can be used to practice nursing skills and/or practice critical thinking while applying medical/nursing knowledge. Medical simulation has been deemed so valuable for students that many state nursing boards allow this time to replace some real patient clinical experiences. If you have the opportunity to attend a nursing school with a simulation center, be sure to take every opportunity of the learning experiences. Be sure to take it seriously – *even though you know the patients are not real.* This time is invaluable because simulation provides faculty the opportunity and time to learn about how you are thinking about the information learned in "the classroom" and help you understand your own thinking process. This helps in the event you need to modify your perspective and understanding of some critical nursing information.

Many adults have a hard time "playing pretend", because we are –adults. This can be the case for faculty and students. The reality is that simulation is a learning opportunity – one of the best and safest. You sometimes do not realize it until after the scenario is over, and begin to discuss the scenarios during the debrief, that there was a deliberate intent for your learning on that day. If you are struggling to "pretend", just give it your best so can still engage in the experiential learning that comes from the debrief discussion. Think about medical simulation like a chemistry or biology lab. The lab helps support and sometimes tests what you have learned in the textbook and in the classroom.

Clinicals

Clinicals...finally! Real patients!

Clinicals are an opportunity to practice learned skills with real patients. This is also the time that you learn a little about the "true" culture of the healthcare environment and nursing. Because there is so much to learn in nursing, use your clinical time wisely. This is the time you receive to apply your knowledge to real patients. When given the opportunity to read through a patient's chart, take the time to actually read through the patient's chart. Do not use this time doing other homework from class. Your faculty will treat you like adults, in hopes that you will take responsibility for your own learning. Reading a patient's chart is more than "just reading". This is the opportunity to look at your patient's many illnesses and medical history and begin putting the pieces together. Your nursing textbook has many small pieces of information in it that you will have to put together someday on your own. Take this time to begin to understand how each piece affects the other. Many hospitals are limiting the number of nursing students that can participate in clinicals at their institution. This is an example of why you should take the clinical experience seriously and learn as much as possible. So, when you get the opportunity, take full advantage of it.

Nursing students are often expected to have a means of transportation due to the clinical requirement. While some nursing schools are located within walking distance to a "university hospital", others may not be. Even if the nursing school is located beside a hospital, you may still be assigned to complete a nursing clinical rotation at another location. Determine what your means of transportation will be prior to beginning nursing school or if one is even required. You must also consider if and how this affects your family; considering you have a family with children while you are in nursing school.

You may wonder how didactics, simulation, and clinicals are related to each other in a nursing program. In general, ONE nursing course *may* be composed of didactic, medical simulation, and clinicals.

Semester 1

Pay attention to detail, be organized, keep up with deadlines and follow instructions. This semester, as with all other semesters, you will learn tons of new information. What you may find most unique about this semester, is that you will learn a new way of reading test questions and taking tests. Yes, in nursing school there are always at least two right answers, and we want you to choose the best answer. When I say, "two right answers", that means that while one of those two answers may seem "right", it will be very "wrong". The best answer means "What is the best intervention for this patient at this very moment – with the information provided?" This can sometimes be a hard fence to climb for those coming into nursing, however, it is a feat that must be overcome. The goal is "critical thinking". If you ever struggled with reading and comprehension of test questions, be sure you begin to work on it early. Start practicing nursing questions and ensure you understand exactly what is being asked. In addition to practicing questions, get in the habit of reading and understanding "rationales" for your correct and incorrect answers. This will help you move forward towards the growth needed to begin thinking like a nurse.

<u>Self-Reflection:</u> What's most unique about nursing school exams, nursing school NCLEX practice exams (HESI & ATI), and nursing boards (NCLEX-RN) is that it is very different from the never-ending standardized exams you experienced in high school. I must say, I was annoyed by the expectation of having to answer so many practice questions in addition to all the other nursing homework/assignments that were required in nursing school. I remember feeling like I was being "tricked" when I answered questions correctly (or so I thought), but they were marked as incorrect. I learned to go to my instructors for understanding, rather than simply asking "why is it wrong?" Although I learned to ask my instructors for help and additional explanations, all the practice questions and wrong answers were still annoying. However, now, having practiced as a nurse, taught nursing students, and have stepped into the physician side of medical education (which is very different from nursing), I have gained new insight on the phrase "critical thinking".

Healthcare is a very rewarding and yet challenging field. The decisions regarding your own healthcare are very much determined by low- and high-level politics. As soon as you begin nursing school, you will begin to hear the phrase "critical thinking" over and over. You will hear it so much that it will begin to sound like a nursing faculty "trend" or "cliché".

It's not until later in your nursing school career that you will realize the importance of thinking differently. Nursing school will not just change the way you think for your patients, but you should be glad to know that it will change the way you assess or view the world around you. Again, your thought process and the way you pay attention to detail will and should change. This is required to be a successful nurse. Should you decide to continue past being a staff RN, you will learn that this type of thinking is required to understand and improve the complex healthcare system – which is part of your responsibility as an RN – improving patient care...globally.

Semester 2 and all other semesters

These semesters will be harder – as they should be. You will learn more information in further detail and may even find yourself questioning information you learned in the previous semester. That is okay. This just means you are thinking – which is what we want you to do. However, whenever possible, always make it a point to understand why there may be differences in information and work with your nursing faculty to determine if those differences are detrimental to your future abilities as a registered nurse, a lack of understanding of the material on your part, or small acceptable differences in caring for a patient per the situation. Remember, in nursing school, no faculty member expects you to remember and know everything, however, you are held responsible for all the information learned in previous semesters. Therefore, it is imperative to utilize every opportunity possible to understand the details and overarching concepts of whatever content you are learning.

Be sure you know how to apply information and make connections between multiple content areas. If you fall behind in the ability to do this, you may suffer when it is time to care for patients and/or take NCLEX-RN – as you are guaranteed to encounter very difficult questions. There may be some questions on the NCLEX-RN that you feel you only understand about 40% or less of the content addressed on that particular question. You should at least be able to conceptually think through the parts of the question you do understand.

How to learn the most during your student clinical rotations

- Be eager to learn
- You will never learn what you have no desire to learn.
- Ask lots of questions

Whether you are working with a patient assigned nurse or a clinical instructor during your clinical rotation, you will begin to realize that you are the only person that is responsible for your learning. That is your job during clinical. The instructor's job is to facilitate your learning and facilitate about seven other students' learning as well. Because your instructor cannot be in eight different places at once, you may spend time with a patient assigned RN. The RN's job is to care for their assigned patients and work with you. You must ask questions and be as resourceful as possible. Some nursing students have had negative clinical experiences because they simply did not take the time to engage in their own learning.

"That nurse doesn't like students"

Remember, your desire to be a nurse is your own desire. Some staff nurses may unintentionally express a lack of care for your desire to be a nurse, and some may even show their distaste for you attempting to be a good nurse because they may perceive that your questions insinuate that they are not good nurses. Some nurses simply do not desire to teach their craft. Everyone did not become a nurse under the impression that they may have to teach someone else about nursing one day – and that is okay. Remember to be professional and tactful with some of your questions when working with staff nurses (non-faculty). You will not encounter this all the time during your clinical rotations, however, there is a good chance you may find yourself working with a nurse that does not appear to be very "nursing student friendly". Remember, that nurses are humans just like everyone else. You should have taken a growth and development course during or prior to nursing school. If you remembered nothing from growth and development, remember that everyone, especially adults have been affected by many aspects and contexts of life. The disgruntled nurse may have experienced something that day or in the distant past or may have forgotten what his/her own experience as a student nurse was like. So, don't be too harsh on those RNs and do not allow them to make you to feel like a burden. However, you should notify your clinical faculty if you run into these issues with a nurse. Again, your desire to be a nurse is your own desire, and you are responsible for fulfilling it.

As a professional of any kind, it your responsibility to take accountable measures for your own learning. What does this mean in clinical? When someone teaches you something in clinical and you don't understand, and don't ask questions, that same someone is still expecting you to be able to successfully complete this task next week (maybe by yourself) – should the opportunity arise.

Always try to keep up

Many educators believe that if you are slowly eased into nursing you will be more successful. This is true in some capacity. You should first determine your learning style and other learning styles you can be flexible in, your breaking point or threshold, and have insight on when you begin to feel completely lost. By knowing this, you can keep yourself from becoming overwhelmed. Unfortunately, with clinical opportunities diminishing across the country, you have got to take every opportunity to learn every minute you are in clinical.

> For example: *If you are in your first semester of nursing school and are just going to your clinical site to obtain vital signs, CBGs, perform bed baths, and complete patient history assessments, there is no reason that you should just be standing around during shift report with no paper and pen. Giving and receiving report is a skill that must be learned. Use that time to practice – even if it is not a "requirement".*

Why does this matter? Ashley, why is this simple message of "keeping up" even being mentioned? Many new nurses have a hard time managing their time and prioritizing care their first year out of nursing school. When provided the opportunity, intellectually engage in your clinical rotation rather than just shadowing your nurse. Once you have begun to master a skill, even in your first semester, consider how you can complete those skills while managing your time appropriately.

Facebook Groups

Some nursing schools have Facebook groups. Some of these groups are organized and updated by the actual nursing school, while others are created and organized by a nursing student for school related social networking. These groups are not always officially associated with the actual nursing school or academic institution. When I was in nursing school, Facebook was not "new", however, we did not use it as a means for communicating to our peers in our nursing program. Today, many nursing students in the same cohort (graduating class) now communicate on Facebook (or other means of social media with discussion boards and/or newsfeeds) about what upcoming assignments have changed, locations for study groups, how to complete assignments or understanding assignment instructions, etc. Today, where being a part of a social media group means you receive a notice when something has been posted, finding ways of connecting with colleagues that have the same academic requirements can be beneficial. These groups can provide reminders and updates that may have slipped your mind during the course of the day or week. However, always remember that Facebook is not a learning management system. What is a learning management system?

A learning management system (LMS) is a software application used to organize your e-learning coursework. These programs are usually organized by each course and contain your graded homework/assignments, projects, rubrics and instructions, quizzes (sometime tests), discussion boards and any other course related information. A couple of examples of an LMS include Blackboard and Moodle. Learning management systems are usually run by your actual nursing school and therefore, you can guarantee the information is reliable.

Always remember, however your academic institution defines the official communication from faculty to student (and vice versa), that is the official form of communication. Period. Any information received from peers on non-official forms of social media may not always be valid, so be sure to check your facts.

A student once told me, in a very disgruntled voice, that she did not submit an assignment or even know about it because it was not posted on Facebook (in their cohort's Facebook group). I was a bit shocked that she even had the audacity to say that to me. I then realized that most adults are so heavily dependent on social media, that it can be easy to forget that Facebook is not an official learning management system and more than likely is not operated by your institution's nursing school.

Should you choose to join any social media group to be connected to your fellow nursing student colleagues, just keep this in mind.

"The nursing school challenge...for all the right reasons."

Things to Remember:

- Nursing school is challenging.
- You will learn a lot about yourself and your peers.
- You will have to work hard.
- Your patients and healthcare team will be depending on you.
- If you haven't already, consider why you like or love nursing...and remember it.

Self-reflection: *One of my positions as an educator has required me to evaluate training at all levels - nursing, physician, etc. While observing an interprofessional (multiple professions learning with and about each other) simulation training, the staff physician faculty stated to the resident physicians ('physicians in training'), "Always remember that your RN is the strongest member on your team." While excited to hear this, I was a bit taken aback, because I wasn't quite sure how this helps the confidence of the residents. He then followed up with the statement, "Your nurses have probably been caring for these types of patients for longer than you have and have encountered many of these similar situations with other physicians. Therefore, when they are providing you with information about the patient and ideas for the care of the patient, you need to be listening." As a nurse educator, this observation made me feel enthusiastic inside about the future of education for healthcare professionals. What you should take away from this statement is that as a RN, your patients and your team are depending you. Therefore, engage in your nursing education so you can learn as much as you can!*

References

This chapter was written 100% from my personal experiences, with no additional resources or references to provide.

Chapter 5: Studying for NCLEX-RN: What to expect

These are some "realistic" expectations that you should have. What to expect…

From a nursing program

Nursing programs are geared towards preparing you to be a nurse that can critically think, be safe, and provide good patient care. All information necessary to be successful on the NCLEX-RN is *usually* provided in your nursing program – in about 6 to 15 different textbooks and over 4-5 semesters.

From a NCLEX-RN prep-course

A prep-course can be a shortened version of everything you have learned in nursing school with the goal of focusing on concepts that will successfully get you through the NCLEX-RN test – without having to re-read 6 to 15 textbooks. The people that teach these courses usually have some "insight" on the way the exam is written and may even be knowledgeable about the common themes of the exam, however, they will not know what exactly is on the exam. They can advance your ability to understand what is being asked in a NCLEX-RN question. They are also able to help you filter your entire nursing program into smaller mental charts that may be easier to mentally reference during the exam.

However, please be advised regarding which type of prep-course you sign up for. There are some courses that focus more of test-taking skills rather than NCLEX-RN content. Some courses will focus on both. Be sure to determine what you are looking for in a prep-course and ensure you are know what you are signing up for.

From yourself

Many academic nurse educators and/or faculty will say to complete 50-75 questions per day to study for NCLEX-RN (some will say more). You must determine what kind of studying practices you have. If you have no intentions of taking a prep-course and are able to stare at your computer to complete 50-75 questions per day, this may be the best option for you. This works well for many people, and others – not so much. If you took a prep-course, and still do not feel confident, and can mentally stand to complete that many questions per day, you should do just that. If extended "screen time" doesn't work for your eyes, hardcopy exam study guides with practice questions can be purchased.

However, if you know that by setting a goal of completing 50-75 questions per day is unrealistic for you, then by continuing with an unrealistic goal, you may be setting yourself up for delaying your NCLEX-RN test date. This can make remembering nursing information even harder – the longer you wait to take NCLEX-RN.

Prep-courses are great, as they can help you make connections between large amounts of nursing information you've learned in the past 2 years. Prep-courses can sometimes even make you feel like "Why did I go to nursing school in first place? I should have just taken a prep-course." Guess what, you will feel that way because nursing school has provided you with a great foundation. (Meaning, you really wouldn't understand the prep-course without nursing school.)

Again, these courses are great, but everyone does not need them. Practice questions are very necessary to prepare your mind for NCLEX-RN type questions. These questions help with learning and better understanding content, but also help with reading and understanding NCLEX type questions. Everyone is different, and studying for NCLEX-RN does not have an attached instructor sending you emails asking you "Why haven't you been studying?", "Why haven't you been applying yourself?" or "Why are you still watching TV?" Therefore, it is solely up to you to determine your own style of studying while considering all the recommendations you will receive – from everyone.

> <u>Self-Reflection</u>: *I met one of my best friends in nursing school. So, of course, when we graduated and needed to study, we were always on the phone watching reality TV – every single day. We were definitely "procrastinators". That's a characteristic that has always been, and still is for me. We graduated in early December and watched TV while talking to each other on the phone until early/mid-January. Daily, while on the phone,*

> *our computers were in our laps, with an intent to study. However, true studying did not occur. I may have read 1-3 pages of information a day and practiced 6-10 questions per day. Once I received the notification that I was "approved to test" and scheduled my exam date, everything became very "real". I had to study like my life depended on it. Not to mention I had already moved to one of the most expensive cities in America – without a job - to be with my fiancé. Therefore, the pressure was on, and I could only afford to take the test once. Seriously, I could only afford one test fee. It was at that point that focusing on studying became easier. Getting off the phone and off social media became easier. I was successful on my 1st attempt in early February.*

This type of study patter or timeline may not work for you. As a matter of fact, I would not even recommend this. However, we all have experienced this type of procrastination at some point in our lives. My biggest recommendation is "don't do what I did". Start early, turn your phone on silent, turn your TV off (or on something you find boring) and start studying as soon as you graduate.

<u>*Additional Resource:*</u> *You can retrieve additional information from the National Council of State Boards of Nursing (NCSBN) site. This will provide you with official information to get you registered appropriately to take the NCLEX-RN. The nursing.org site can provide you additional information about studying for NCLEX-RN.*

References

National Council of State Boards of Nursing, Inc. (2018). Before the exam. Retrieved from https://www.ncsbn.org/

Nursing.org. (2018). Overcoming the NCLEX. Retrieved from https://www.nursing.org/resources/nclex/

Chapter 6: Landing your first position

"There's a huge nursing shortage!!!"

Writing your resume

Details, details, details!

Many new and experienced nurses believe that a short resume or curriculum vitae (CV) is great because it has just enough information on it without burdening the reader with all the details about your experience. While this may be very true, this also allows for a false depiction of your experience and/or a misunderstanding of your experience. I have chaired and sat on interview committees where I've watched colleagues *guess* someone's experiences because details were not present (these applicants followed the application instructions and submitted a one-page CV – rather than a detailed CV). If you can clearly demonstrate your professional work, experience, publications, awards and successes through highlights "only", one page may work for you, but I doubt it. When applying for your first nursing job, often your only nursing experience is described by your clinical rotations.

You will see that I use the words CV and resume interchangeably. They do not mean the same thing; however, the point is that whatever you submit, be sure it has "the details".

The federal government has a universal website for all individuals seeking federal employment. This website is also used for nurses that are seeking federal employment. Many of the nursing positions posted to this site have a statement that says this (or something very similar): *In describing your experience, please be clear and specific. We may not make assumptions regarding your experience.* Hence, what does this mean for you? This means (in my opinion) that if it is not on your resume, do not get upset when your resume does not get forwarded to hiring officials. Also, keep in mind that if a pediatric job opening states specific abilities they are looking for, do not assume they know you have experience in those areas just because your resume says "Pediatric Ward Nurse" under the work experience section. Add the details.

Your resume will determine whether you get offered "the golden ticket" ...an interview. Before anyone even meets you, they see your resume or CV. While you may be able to knock socks off at the interview, you should really be knocking socks off the recipients of your resume or CV first. During the interview is when you knock the rest of their clothes off!

If you feel like you have accomplished great things during your capstone or preceptorship experience (in nursing school), don't discount it. If you have healthcare related volunteer experience in the community, at your neighbors' home, at church, etc., don't discount it! Add it to your resume!

Should I get a medical-surgical job first?

"Get a year or two of med-surg experience under your belt and you should be fine wherever you go." ...Maybe...maybe not

Advantages

- You are guaranteed to obtain a plethora of great nursing experience on a med-surg floor.
- You will learn a way of nursing and managing very chronically ill patients like none other.
- There are often more jobs – especially for new graduate nurses – in med-surg areas, as compared to other areas in healthcare.
- You will maintain certain competencies learned in school that you may lose in other areas.

Disadvantages

- There is no absolute guarantee that working on a med-surg floor will make you a better ICU, peds, OR, or other type of nurse.
- If you have a true passion for another nursing specialty, such as Labor and Delivery, you will have a hard time enjoying "nursing" when waking up to go to work every day to a med-surg floor.

In any job that requires large amounts of physical, mental, and emotional efforts from the employee, it is almost imperative that the employee enjoys what they do and the environment in which they do it. Consider this when applying to nurse positions.

Interview time

Dress: Not too much time will be spent here. No skin! If you are even questioning if a clothing article is appropriate for an interview, don't wear it. If you look in the mirror and you "look good", you may want to re-evaluate your outfit to ensure it does not look like you are headed to a nightclub. If you look in the mirror, and you can barely move, don't wear it. If you look in the mirror and are dazzled by your jewelry, don't wear it. If you look in the mirror and you see absolutely nothing wrong, you may lack all insight of how to dress for an interview. Lastly, if you look in the mirror and you look "smart, conservative, innovative, and intuitive", that outfit is probably the best choice. What does that outfit look like? Well, sometimes, you just know! This just might be the most SUBJECTIVE paragraph in this book. It may even be relatively confusing, as there is no definitive answer to what appropriate dress looks like, however, the point of this paragraph is... be yourself, but do not go into an interview looking crazy.

Communication: Do I really need to address this? Please learn how to talk at an interview. Don't be cocky. "I" should usually be "we". "I" should be used when discussing your leadership abilities and then followed with "we" when discussing the team that you led. Be respectful. This section should not even be here, however, I recognize that sometimes we all need reminders.

Inexperienced: Some people believe that because you lack decades of nursing experience, you are not qualified for a job. Let them think that. However, you should not think that way – don't sell yourself short. In nursing, life experience can be a great attribute – in addition to your nursing experience. Depending on your age, some interviewers may even believe that not only do you lack nursing experience, but you even lack life experience or technology. Do not let that get you stuck in an interview. Be prepared to provide ALL your experience and explain how it applies to the job you are interviewing for. Never sell yourself short because of what you think the interviewer/s want to hear. While you may not have exactly what they want to hear, realize that you do have life experience handling challenging situations. Pull from what you have.

Answering questions properly*:* Whether you realize it or not, there is a right and a wrong way to answer all interview questions. You should always provide an example through explanation. If the example you provided was of a problem, be sure to explain the steps you took to resolve this problem. I would even recommend this type question answering for yes or no questions – just make the description very brief. This type of question answering is primarily necessary for "Problem Based Interviewing", however, I would recommend you answer interview questions like these during any interview – even when it doesn't feel like the questions were written to obtain very much information from you. The VA often engages in problem-based interviewing, and they provide more information about it on their website.

Some interviews will begin by letting you know they have a busy schedule interviewing multiple people back to back. This means they are pressed for time. Be sure to answer the questions thoroughly and be concise.

Be sure to always provide an answer. Draw on all nursing experiences, volunteer experience, and sometimes even life experience. However, if you feel confident in your previous responses and genuinely do not have an answer for a particular question, "winging it" may not be the best choice. You may want to say, "At this time I cannot think of an example where I have experienced this exact situation, however, should I encounter it, I believe I would..." (Be clear and concise).

Nursing shortage - seriously?

How does one truly answer this question?

Without talking about healthcare goals and all these other large national and organizational studies that show the increased and continuously increasing need for RNs in healthcare, yes, there is a nursing shortage. HOWEVER, …the big however…

Changing the culture of healthcare is hard! Healthcare is so dynamic. With so many requirements of healthcare professionals regarding school, credentials, day to day expectations when caring for patients, expectations of hospitals, expectations of hospital leadership, accrediting bodies, increasing patient needs, etc., changing these environments is more than a challenge. Some may even say it's nearly impossible – no matter how many regulations come down on hospitals. *What does this have to do with a nursing shortage? Everything.*

A nursing shortage – what exactly does this mean? Does this mean individuals with RN credentials? Does this mean some individuals with RN credentials and some with LVN credentials? Does this mean individuals with RN credentials that are able to manage the growing expectations of the RN during a given shift? What does "quality care" actually mean? If there are enough RNs (numerically) on "my" floor, why do I need to hire more? When I am looking at FTEs, am I looking at "quality" or "quantity"? Am I looking at the time spent maneuvering through policies or the lack there of in order to provide "quality" patient care? What does quality have to do with me having to spend money on a new nurse when I have "enough" FTEs?

Having been a new nurse not too long ago (about seven years ago), I have an appreciation for the belief that "because of the nursing shortage" I will get a RN position immediately after nursing school. Unfortunately, this is just not the case.

If you are a new nurse, hospitals are "taking a risk" hiring you (as with any job). However, in a hospital, sick patients don't "stop getting sick". Production cannot stop due to your inexperience. Financially, many facilities prefer hiring people with experience in the specialty area. This means less training days (training days = paying two people for the same shift), and increased chance of retention due to the fact that the new employee is more likely to have job satisfaction, when they are applying for a position they have worked before. (Although, even hiring an experienced nurse is a risk.) The 2018 National Healthcare Retention & RN Staffing Report states that a hospital can lose between $4.4 million and $7.0 million annually due to staff nurse turnover. About 17.5% of new nurses leave their first job within 1 year of starting their jobs (Kovner, et al, 2014).

These numbers are somewhat alarming and an example to why some employers have a hard time opening some "New Graduate Nurse Programs" for applications during graduation season.

What generation do you fall in? Do you believe in having a work-life balance? No matter your age, you may be striving for a work-life balance. Progressive organizations often agree in the ideals of having a positive work-life balance; however, this benefit can be challenging to provide with the ever-increasing patient needs/illnesses and hospital, government, and accrediting organizational demands.

Keep in mind, going into healthcare to help save lives is not like working at a car shop. While the customers are still humans, and their bodies are constantly changing at a faster rate than our world and technology can keep up with in healthcare. Some people choose to go into nursing because of the "the promise of a guaranteed job" while others go into nursing with the desire to help people. Think about why you chose nursing and use that to keep you going when you are pressing forward to find a job.

All in all, yes there is a nurse shortage. Just remember, that does not mean that the jobs are going to be waiting for you. If you are a new nurse, you cost a large amount of money, and you could cost even more if you are "not feeling the job". You will have to sell yourself and your abilities. Consider also selling your unique abilities of fresh thinking and using evidence to enhance your practice as a nurse.

What are your plans for the future?

Are you hoping to go back to school? You may want to consider institutions that are willing to pay for you to go back to school. Simply keep in mind that there is usually some kind of time commitment required when an organization or institution pays for you to go back to school.

Are planning on moving? Are you willing to move? If so, where? Is staying with the same organization important to you? If so, will your job be able to transfer to the new location? These are all questions to be thinking about when planning your future and even applying to jobs.

Waiting forever to get a job offer...or even an interview?

Things to consider:

- This may be the norm at the time you are graduating from nursing school.
- Were there any staff nurse vacancies on the floor you performed your preceptorship (or your last nursing student clinical rotation)? If so, speak to that nurse manager.
- Have you considered going into the military?
- Are you mobile? Are you able to move to another area/location? If so, this could open your position opportunities significantly.

References

Kovner, C. T., Brewer, C. S., Fatehi, F., & Jun, J. (2014). What Does Nurse Turnover Rate Mean and What Is the Rate? *Policy, Politics, & Nursing Practice*, *15*(3–4), 64–71. https://doi.org/10.1177/1527154414547953

Nursing Solutions, Inc., National Healthcare Retention & RN Staffing Report. (2018). Report of the *2018 National Healthcare Retention & RN Staffing Report*. Retrieved from http://www.nsinursingsolutions.com/files/assets/library/retention-institute/nationalhealthcarernretentionreport2018.pdf

Chapter 7: Generational expectations and biases

Most people will not be honest with you about this or sometimes lack insight to see it, however, I – as always – will be honest about it!

While generational expectations, biases, and stereotypes should not exist...they do, and most of the time, the leadership making decisions are often of the generation or generations before you. Keep in mind; this is *not always* the case – as I have worked with great supervisors and colleagues of previous generations (meaning older than I). However, within these same workplaces, I have also worked with many colleagues (on hiring committees) that have made statements about my generation – not knowing how old I was at the time. If you are preparing for "interview time" then you have already learned that as nurses, we should not stereotype people; every single human being is different and comes from different contexts of life. However, nurses are good at "assessing" their patients. We are just spectacular at this!

With this being said, I plan to address some of the bias realities that exist in some workplaces.

"Empowered thinking"

There are many that believe that younger generations often feel a sense of entitlement or feeling empowered. There are also many that use this word or phrase incorrectly and without full understanding.

Sometimes when I hear this word, it's used to describe individuals of particularly younger generations. It is often used when referring to students, applicants or employees that are simply not willing to work hard, are not knowledgeable about how to be professional as it relates to proper communication to supervisors or instructors, or simply lack the ability to take accountability for their poor decisions. Now, really these people may just be called "lazy" or "unprofessional". The word "empowered" or "entitled" comes into play when these same individuals still expect "success" or "advancement" in their student or work life. Now this is what I would call the negative stigma that is often seen and heard when the words "empowered generation" are mentioned. Unfortunately, you only have to live a little to realize that there are many people from every generation that function in this manner. So, while I believe it's of poor taste and understanding and an unfortunate situation when this "title" is placed only on younger generations, you should know that this exists.

Also know that I feel a little different about the word "empowered generation". Some generations – like mine – were raised during a time where the idea of going to school to obtain a high-level degree was the best thing to do. However, when those generations got out of school (college), the economy barely had jobs for them and tuition costs in this country had already begun to sky-rocket prior to graduation. Therefore, these generations have and still *expect* some type of return on investment for the time and money put into earning these high-level degrees – as any sane human would *expect*. I believe this is simply an unfortunate economic situation that creates automatic stereotyping of individuals – often based on their age.

Regardless, of where you fall within the negative stereotypes of younger generations, know that this stereotyping does exist in some places. However, also know that no matter your age, it is okay to feel empowered - as there is a positive connotation to that word – and it is okay to maintain high expectations for the life you want to live. Just be sure to always remain professional.

<u>Ready to Retire</u>

"Not him, he's gonna make us repost this position next year. You do know how long it took to get this position approved through HR, right?"

This is another generational statement heard while reviewing resumes and discussing interview results. This statement is often referring to the RN that has made nursing their new career at a later age. Whether you, the RN, are looking for your first, second, third, or last position, someone is always looking at finances and time. Many things in our country are driven by money – healthcare is one of them. It cost money to hire you, to train you, and to lose you – no matter your age. Unfortunately, there is an assumption that if you are of a "certain age", you will only be working "for but so long". This doesn't even include the "physical assessment" of bodily functions that occurs during nursing interviews. Remember, we are always "assessing".

What are you talking about Ashley!?!

I'm referring to the fact that while your age may not be determined by your resume, someone may be determining it during your interview. Someone is potentially assuming that because of your age, you may only be able to physically function at a certain level when caring for patients. The reality is that you and your resume should be on the same playing field as anyone else's. However, recognizing that this bias exists is only the first step. Now you need to work around it. It doesn't make it right but ignoring it doesn't help either. For example, it is not required that you put your high school graduation date, or every work experience you have ever had on your resume – especially when it is not relevant. Once you get to your interview, always have goals! Your goals should be related to growth within the organization you are hoping to work for. Those goals should say, "I am not leaving tomorrow" – even if you decide to leave next week.

Unprofessional Dress

Why are you talking about this again Ashley?!

Because you must understand how this is sometimes linked with generational biases. While I haven't heard many comments about expectations of how an interviewee will dress prior to the actual interview, I have definitely heard generational comments immediately after an interviewee walked out the interview. Be informed, you can have the best interview ever, answer the questions perfectly, etc., but if you show up to an interview dressed unprofessionally, there is a good chance that you may not be hired by a generationally biased or non-biased committee. I have witnessed this first hand. A great candidate left the room once, and the next statement made was, "She is not mature enough for this job. Did you see her shirt? Her cleavage?" While the truth of the matter is that cleavage does not directly determine levels of maturity, it can make a difference in many professional environments – so just dress professionally... please.

Generation biases are real. You would be surprised how serious this can be. The example I will describe is truly from experience. Imagine having a relatively older female candidate come in with cleavage showing, and the female interviewer discuss this lady as "professional" and spoke only of her verbal responses during the interview. However, when the same female interviewer discussed another younger female candidate with the same amount of cleavage showing, the discussion was focused on her cleavage and her appearance – not her verbal responses...

When you are trying to get a job, you will not be able to remove generational biases. Your primary job is to overcome the limitations associated with these biases. I do not believe in modifying who you are because of stereotypes that exists, however, the reality is ...they unfortunately exist, and you need a job. You must first recognize these biases exist and then be sure to make yourself marketable no matter your audience. If this reality bothers you, "get in" and change it from the inside. Truthfully, if you are a professional person period, this should not affect you too much.

Additional Resources: *Below are two articles that discuss generations, generational biases, and even mention some feelings related to generational biases. This chapter and these articles do not excuse generational biases, they just show that the biases exist.*

- ✓ *Multi-generational impacts on the workplace*
- ✓ *Age-based stereotypes: a major cause of inter-generational tension*

References

Achieve Global. (2011). *Age-based stereotypes: a major cause of inter-generational tension*. (Business Issue). Tampa, FL: Perrin, C.

Center for Women and Business at Bentley University. (2017). *Multi-generational impacts on the workplace* (Curated Research Report). Retrieved from Bentley University, Center for Women and Business website: https://www.bentley.edu/files/2017/11/01/Bentley%20CWB%20Generational%20Impacts%20Research%20Report%20Fall%202017.pdf

Chapter 8: First year working as an RN

Myths and Truths

Myth #1: "Don't worry, they will train you; they won't just throw you out there."

Truth #1: While many facilities have transition-to-practice programs or residency programs, there is no guarantee that any or every facility will fully prepare you for what is in store when you are fully responsible for your own full load of patients. There will be a learning curve when you begin working as a registered nurse. It is your responsibility to recognize it and speak up when you realize you are missing information about something. This is not to say that you will receive "no" preparation. Just do not think that you can ever be "fully" prepared or that an institution can support the "preparation" of one RN (financially) until you are "fully prepared".

Myth #2: "Employers want to improve patient outcomes and want you to be a positive change agent."

Truth #2: Employers want to improve patient outcomes – yes. However, oftentimes new graduates have high level expectations of positive change in healthcare facilities based on what was learned in nursing school about change agents, patient advocacy, and evidence-based practice (EBP). Remember that change is a slow process. You may encounter MANY barriers, but don't give up, don't stress, and try not to change the culture of a unit or a hospital facility in one day. This will not only wear you down, it may negatively impact your relationships with direct leadership and potentially your peers. This breakdown of relationships in a work environment can create a hostile work environment. Your job is to make it through your first year.

Many nurses and other professionals may not agree with this honesty. But it is true. You can try to bust down doors with all your EBP knowledge and energy and then fall apart after realizing that you are not successful in any capacity. Or you can realize that culture change takes time. Sometimes it's best to work on this change in teams that already exist. Be sure not to allow a broken system to cause compassion fatigue. This can happen to anyone – sometimes when you don't even realize it (Sheppard, 2016). It has happened to me! *The High Cost of Nurse Turnover* (University of New Mexico, 2016) discusses mental, emotional, and physical demands of nursing. This article is great because it is a quick read and simplifies nursing and healthcare in a few short sections. Nursing comes with many demands and many rewards. Be sure to take care of yourself by giving your best, while recognizing that healthcare is not perfect, but slowly moving in the right direction.

Myth #3: "You will learn your facility's policies and unit policies regarding procedures and nurse expectations when you begin working."

Truth #3: Yes, you will learn many of your facility's policies during orientation classes, transition-to-practice class, residency classes, and/or on-the floor training, however, you will not learn all the policies during this time. You will still be held responsible, however, for all the facility's policies. Therefore, take responsibility in being resourceful in how to handle certain situations and be resourceful and proactive when your nursing judgement calls something to question.

Myth #4: "It is normal for a physician (or primary care provider) or a nurse to scream, curse, and be sarcastic or rude when you call or speak to them."

Truth #4: This is not a normal occurrence. It may or may not be frequent depending on the individual or institution but should not be described as "normal". This is also not acceptable. If you ever find this to be a normal occurrence in any facility, it is very unfortunate and probably means that the culture in that particular facility is so complacent with this behavior, that nurses probably do not feel supported or empowered enough to speak up about having to function in a hostile work environment – which, by the way, is a type of harassment.

Will you ever encounter this or something similar? Probably. However, as with any work environment, handle "urgent" situations NOW. Address inappropriate & disrespectful behavior in the appropriate manor – sometimes that means handling it a bit later. Always follow the chain of command...and yes, this means to start with the inappropriate/disrespectful individual the first time this happens.

Additional Resource: In 2016, the Joint Commission issued "Bullying has no place in health care". This is a great document and a good read for all healthcare workers. I like this document because when it comes to "harassment", the victim is often trying to ensure they meet the qualifications to say, "I feel harassed." Most labor laws discuss forms of harassment; however, do not quite define it in a way that is relatable to a healthcare employee (my personal opinion). There are additional resources at the end of this chapter that are very interesting as well.

Myth #5: "You will be able to leave your job feeling good about yourself because you are helping people."

Truth #5: You will, however, remember that you can't save everyone, and that's okay. Healthcare can't save everyone. As a matter of fact, you may find that you were only able to barely help 1 out of the 15 things that a patient needs fixing. You may even go home some days or nights feeling like crap, because you realize there is only so much you can do to help a patient and their family because you finally realize the sad truth - we live in a capitalistic world that only moves for the dollar and many of your patients have comorbidities (therefore, they are expensive). Remember, the phrase "improving patient outcomes" is not referring to the patient you are caring for "that day". It's referring to patients globally - as a whole...over a period of time. You may also find that many healthcare facilities/systems are so broken, and function very differently than your nursing textbook discussed as best practice. This can be frustrating. Do not give up, however, do not allow it to wear you down. Understand your environment and understand your environment's motivation for change. Remember, even one small improvement to patient care or a patient's life can positively affect many aspects of life and dimensions around you.

Myth #6: "Nursing can be a stressful underpaid public servant type job."

Truth #6: Nursing, as with other public servant positions, is what you make it. I strongly believe in the idea of choosing a career and a position that makes you happy. When starting any job, you will spend a significant amount of time learning the ropes. However, you should be happy doing what you are doing. Nursing can be a very rewarding field for many reasons. One beauty of nursing is that it has *so many* directions whenever you are too stressed and/or ready for a change. I will never forget my nursing instructor's comment in nursing school. We both witnessed a rude nurse grumbling under her breath about a patient. My nursing instructor said, "She is probably a great nurse. Unfortunately, she might be so worn down, that her attitude is affecting her patient care. The best thing she can do is move into another area of nursing where she can be happy." Now, out of nursing school, I agree with that statement entirely. You are not "running away" or giving up when you decide to leave. Once you cannot control your emotions, you must reconsider your current situation – for yourself and for your patients.

Pushing through what you don't know

Take responsibility for your own learning.

In nursing, you will never learn or be taught everything you need to know about *nursing* – there is simply too much to learn from a textbook and too much to learn from experience. Some of the learning will come from your first job as a nurse. On your first job, or any other subsequent job, be honest about what you are not comfortable with – there are people's lives at hand. However, be willing and ready to learn what you don't know. After being taught something, be sure you understand it and the rationale and evidence behind it. The next time you encounter the same situation, you may not be perfect at handling this same situation, but you should be knowledgeable. Be resourceful and look back at any old notes or the facility's resources, policies, procedure steps, etc. to refresh your memory, if necessary. Again, perfection is not key to success. Preceptors and managers want to know you have a desire and drive to learn and have the ability to retain and apply information learned from written resources *and* previous experiences.

Shared Governance

If there are opportunities to be a part of a committee or team on your unit or within your hospital facility, be sure to join! Because the time on these committees will/should ultimately contribute to "improving patient outcomes", you are technically still working. Therefore, you should still get paid for this time. Being a part of these committees and teams not only gives you and your nursing colleagues a voice in decision making, it also provides you the opportunity to meet people, have people meet you, allow people in leadership & hiring roles to see your presence, work ethic, critical thinking abilities and dedication to the organization. These opportunities assist in learning more about what is going on in your facility and how the decisions are derived. This also looks great on your resume when applying to another nurse position. On your resume, this shows recruiters and nurse managers that you are knowledgeable about more than just staff nursing.

Friendships do not have to occur with every colleague

Everyone will not like you...and that is A-Okay! Hopefully you did not decide on a nursing career to have everyone in the world like you. Remember back in middle school or high school where you had only a few *real* friends and everyone else was simply...everyone else. There were even people that blatantly couldn't stand you. Well guess what, welcome back. You can expect this type of environment in any work place setting – especially if your colleagues are humans. The biggest difference is how you handle and deal with the people that do not like you. You are no longer in middle and high school; therefore, expectations of more mature and professional responses are present. You have probably already learned that no matter the situation, you are a nurse and you are expected to be professional even in hard situations. Sometimes, however, you may not realize how these situations can affect you internally when you leave from work. You must first recognize that a certain someone is causing you grief – simply from just working with them. It may not always be the "entire system" or the "entire work environment". Once you realize who this person is, learn how to professionally deal and work with this person. It's easier to deal with these types of people after you first recognize their behaviors are their personality and may not change; rather than allowing it to always catch you off guard. Also, keep in mind that these behaviors may change if you professionally approach the person – as they may not be aware of their own attitude, demeanor, or your perception of their attitude.

Most importantly, learn how to deal with difficult people in a way that does not affect you too much. They are everywhere in hospitals/healthcare, as a hospital is often a high stress environment.

References

Gillespie, G. L., Grubb, P. L., Brown, K., Boesch, M. C., & Ulrich, D. (2017). "Nurses Eat Their Young": A Novel Bullying Educational Program for Student Nurses. *Journal of nursing education and practice*, *7*(7), 11-21.

Lombardo, B. & Eyre, C. (2011). Compassion fatigue: A nurse's primer. *The Online Journal of Issues in Nursing*. 16(1). doi: 10.3912/OJIN.Vol16No01Man03

Sheppard, K. (2016, January). Compassion fatigue: Are you at risk? *American Nurse Today*, 11(1), 53-55.

The Joint Commission. (2016). Bullying has no place in health care (Quick Safety Issue 24). Retrieved from Division of Health Care Improvement website: https://www.jointcommission.org/assets/1/23/Quick_Safety_Issue_24_June_2016.pdf

The University of New Mexico. (2016). The high cost of nurse turnover. Retrieved from https://rnbsnonline.unm.edu/articles/high-cost-of-nurse-turnover.aspx

Chapter 9: Nurses vs Doctors

We are sooooooo DIFFERENT...aren't we?

As with any environment that requires socialization, healthcare has different groups of professionals often working, living, eating, and sleeping "alongside" another group. Outside of the hospital or healthcare environment, this can be described as "coexisting". We often see the "coexist" bumper stickers on people's cars and there is often a perceived positive connotation associated with it. However, healthcare professionals coexisting is not appropriate when it comes to caring for patients. It's simply not enough.

<u>Why describe it this way?</u>

Unfortunately, I have heard statements made by some professions about other professions that clearly show a lack of understanding of one another. These types of misunderstandings create barriers and can often make it challenging to provide collaborative care to patients (working together as a team to care for patients). The Interprofessional Education Collaborative (IPEC) is an effort initiated by a group of multiple healthcare professionals. Their focus is discussing the need for interprofessional education to promote collaborative practice. In healthcare there are often a group of professionals that are supposed to be working together to care for patients. This should be the case every time a patient walks into a healthcare environment. However, because of some "coexisting" environments, the care that is being provided is very fragmented.

> _Self-Reflection_: *I attended a spectacular five-day world-renowned training for different types of healthcare professionals – with most of the attendees being physicians. Towards the end of this training week, we began to discuss interprofessional education. There clearly was no intent to dive into the nuts and bolts of interprofessional education per the IPEC, however, we were slotted time to address the thoughts and feelings behind certain professions. One of the statements made by a nurse practitioner (an attendee) was that nurses often feel like they are treated like they are of a lower socioeconomic status. The actual description used was "second class citizens". When this statement was made, I was so glad it was said. This is often what I have seen, experienced, and heard stories about. However, when the floor was initially opened for an interprofessional education discussion, I was uncertain as to how this could be expressed in the training we were in (with majority of the attendees being physicians). Interprofessional education is my absolute*

passion and felt relatively biased about its value, so I wanted to sit back and listen to others' thoughts. What was great about this course was that nurses and physicians do not often get to work together to be honest about their feelings, experiences, and thoughts regarding healthcare cultures and environments. The venue and structure of the course created vulnerabilities for everyone, which allowed a deeper level of honesty amongst all the participants.

Most of my nursing career has been spent socializing with other nurses. What does this mean exactly? Most of my time "not providing direct patient care" has been spent with other nurses. Therefore, up until now, I only had the opportunity to hear from and relate to other nurses. This often creates a disillusion that nurses are the *only* health professionals dealing with certain types of healthcare professional relationship stressors – horizontal violence, hierarchy, peer pressure, titles, ranks, etc. These types of misunderstandings promote an unfortunate and often unrecognizable distaste for certain other professions that may be perceived as not experiencing the same stressors. This disillusion can sometimes even begin in nursing school.

Let's examine how we (nursing) propagate this type of thinking – *all seen first-hand*:

Nursing schools must hire adjunct clinical nurse faculty in order to survive. These adjuncts may or may not have a thorough understanding of the curriculum and teachings of the home institution from which the student attends. These adjuncts also work with 5-8 nursing students at a time. Therefore, not only are the nursing students working with adjunct faculty, they are also potentially working with other non-teaching experienced/developed registered nurses that have the ability to implant socialization cultures that do not promote interprofessional collaboration. This is not always the case, but do remember the concept "compassion fatigue"? This was mentioned and referenced in Chapter 7. Compassion fatigue can be displaced to those you are mentoring. It's effects not only trickle down to patients, but a preceptor or faculty's compassion fatigue can sometimes affect student perceptions of healthcare interpersonal relationships.

> <u>Self-Reflection</u>: *When I was in my last year of nursing school, I had two preceptors for the same rotation. Having two preceptors allowed me to get my required clinical hours in for that semester. The two had different styles of nursing and different styles of teaching. The differences were very helpful for me in choosing my own "style of nursing". These differences also helped me to learn more about nursing, as I receive different perspective on how to accomplish the same goals. There were some differences that made me a bit uncomfortable sometimes. One of my preceptors would use the phrase "baby docs". While this phrase does not sound harmful, it is often used when describing a junior physician (or junior physician resident) that may not be as "compliant" as a nurse would like them to be. Notice I didn't say this phrase is often used*

when describing a junior physician (or junior physician resident). What I found even more interesting, is that during some of our program's required monthly meetings, I could tell that my peers (fellow students) were learning some of these phrases as well.

Your new graduate nurse program is stellar! While the nurses that have been mentoring, precepting, and nurturing you through the adjustment process have been great, you have still spent all your time with nurses only.

Oftentimes, the only down to earth, non-patient related conversations you will have with physicians are the cynical jokes made in passing. There is not enough time in the day for a physician to spend as much time with a staff nurse as a staff nurse spends with another staff nurse.

Fortunately for me, I recently have had the opportunity to spend 40-hour weeks learning about physician residency education, cultures, and other experiences that affect physicians. I will never be able to say I fully understand what it means to be a physician, but I never would have thought there was so much about their experience as they grow during their career that I didn't know. Many of my thoughts about the differences between nurses and physicians – learned during my time being socialized as a nurse – have now all gone out the window. There are a few things that are true, while most are simply misunderstood. We, as nurses, tend to believe we are the "vulnerable" profession in healthcare. Resident physicians, junior physicians, and other healthcare professionals are also vulnerable to the same experiences we have – just in different ways. They are stressed. They experience levels of hierarchy and rank when making decisions. They experience fear of perceptions of incompetence when they ask for help, not due to actual incompetence, but due to unprofessional retribution for deferring to an expert in the best interest of the patient. They want to help patients as much as you do, but often feel the same pressures you feel by the healthcare systems. These pressures often make it feel like the healthcare system wants you to do everything but help patients.

I say all of this to say, do not prejudge physicians, or any other healthcare profession. Take what you hear about them with a grain of salt, and professionally get to know them – if possible. If you do not get a chance to do this, at least take the time to read articles about the stressors physicians and other professions are dealing with. You may find that you can communicate with them better and vice versa when you both understand each other a little better. Mostly, change the culture of nursing by changing the way you socialize another new nurse or nursing student – saving the negative subjective comments for.... yourself.

References

Interprofessional Education Collaborative Expert Panel. (2011). *Competencies for Interprofessional Collaborative Practice: Report of an expert panel.* Washington, D.C.

Lombardo, B. & Eyre, C. (2011). Compassion fatigue: A nurse's primer. *The Online Journal of Issues in Nursing*. 16(1). doi: 10.3912/OJIN.Vol16No01Man03

Sheppard, K. (2016, January). Compassion fatigue: Are you at risk? *American Nurse Today*, 11(1), 53-55.

Chapter 10: Certification & going back to school

I want some ALPHABET SOUP!

Why get certified?

Getting certified enhances your career by distinguishing you from other RNs or other professionals and shows your ability and dedication to providing excellent care. It is often recognized by colleagues and employers as a way of dedicating yourself to a specialty or specialties in nursing.

Some institutions provide incentive awards for specializing, while others offer payment for the certification exam and an incentive award. Some institutions offer no assistance with the exam costs and offer no incentive award. You must decide the motivation behind getting certified. If you know you will be applying for another job at some point, your certification credentials may help you obtain your next position and/or increase your salary for your next position.

Certification Organizations

There are many certification organizations and certification types. Some certifications require time spent working on a certain type of floor/unit prior to being eligible to sit for the certification exam. Other certification types require both education in a specific nursing field *and* time spent working in that area prior to exam eligibility. Some only require education in a nursing specialty. Think about what you would like to be certified in and/or what certification exam you are eligible to sit for. Lippincott NursingCenter's *Nursing Certification Boards by Specialty* (2019) offers a thorough list of potential nursing certifications by specialty and includes organization contact information. You would be surprised to know of the many nursing opportunities that exist.

Going Back to School

What options are out there and what's the difference?

Nursing Focused Options include MSN, DNP, and PhD. Nursing Focused means the degree will be another nursing degree. They usually require a previous nursing degree and will result with an advance degree in a specialty area having to do with nursing.

You are probably like "Duh!" Well, healthcare systems are very dynamic, so of course advancing in healthcare degrees is now very dynamic as well! "What are you talking about Ashley?" Thanks for asking! Continue reading!

Non-Nursing Focused Options include: MS and PhD. Non-Nursing Focused graduate degrees are those that focus on improving healthcare and/or healthcare systems without requiring a nursing background prior to being in that graduate program. These programs may offer very similar curriculum and be titled the same as the nursing focused graduate programs, but they are not offered through the "Nursing Department" or "School/College of nursing". They may be offered through the "Nursing Department" but are open for non-nursing students.

Examples of Nursing & Non-Nursing Focused programs that are similar (this is not all inclusive):

[MSN → Master of Science in Nursing; MS → Master of Science]

- MSN in Nursing Informatics vs MS in Healthcare Informatics
- MSN Healthcare Administration & Management vs. MS in Healthcare Administration
- PhD in Nursing Informatics vs PhD in Healthcare Informatics
- MSN in Community/Public Health vs. MS Public Health

<u>Why are these programs so similar and which do I choose?</u>

The healthcare environment is ever changing. The one thing that has not and will not change is that there is always room for improvement in the care that is delivered. Improved care often comes from improved processes and increasing quantity and quality of the providers at all levels and specialties. There is truly a shortage in many areas of healthcare. Having multiple pathways to improving care creates options for those interested in healthcare as a profession.

There are always advantages and disadvantages to choosing one program over the other (nursing focused vs non-nursing focused). A huge consideration to be made is your plan for the future regarding becoming an educator of nurses. Most nursing schools at all levels require at least a Master of Science in NURSING (no matter the focus). If you do not have this requirement, you may be required to at least have a PhD or DNP (one of the terminal degrees).

This requirement may only affect you if you have no intentions of obtaining a terminal degree (doctorate degree). For example, if you have a BSN and a MS in Healthcare Informatics, some institutions might say that you are not qualified to teach nursing students. Whereas the nurse with the BSN, and the MSN in Nursing Informatics would qualify. What in the world!?!? This comes from nursing school accreditation requirements. Some schools function differently, but you should be mindful that this does happen.

What about obtaining a terminal degree? PhD or DNP – which is better?

This is a topic that always comes up when discussing nursing terminal degrees. The conversation often focuses on one being better than the other. One is more accepted than the other. One degree has requirements that are "easier" to fulfill than the other. One degree requires you to become an advanced practice nurse first (nurse practitioner) or at least become one during the program. THIS INFORMATION IS NOT TRUE. Your decision to apply for a DNP or PhD program should be dependent on your nursing career goals – and maybe even the type of student you are. Doctor of Philosophy (PhD) programs are often research-focused programs whose graduates typically teach and/or conduct research. Doctor of Nursing Practice (DNP) programs often focus on clinical practice or leadership roles.

When deciding on a program (PhD or DNP), be sure to read the curriculum for each program and each focus track. There was a time when becoming a DNP required that you be a nurse practitioner first. This is no longer the case. There was a time when if you were not a nurse practitioner and interested in getting a DNP, you would still have to go through nurse practitioner curriculum to fulfill DNP curricular requirements. This is also no longer the case. You can now obtain a DNP with or without becoming a nurse practitioner. There are also more pathways to obtaining a DNP and more focus areas when obtaining a PhD. So, again, be sure to read through the curriculum, the backgrounds of the faculty that teach in those programs and think about how you would like to utilize the degrees in your practice. Each option will provide you the opportunity to teach – should you so choose to.

Additional Resources: There are two articles that discuss in detail the PhD and DNP educational pathways and discusses the past issues, present issues, and considerations for the future. These are good reads! Additional information for how to locate these are in the references section.

- ✓ *A critical examination of developments in nursing doctoral education in the United States*
- ✓ *Choosing a pathway: PhD or DNP?*

References

Ketefian, S., & Redman, R. W. (2015). A critical examination of developments in nursing doctoral education in the United States. *Revista latino-americana de enfermagem, 23*(3), 363-71.

Lippincott NursingCenter (2019). *Nursing Certification Boards by Specialty.* Retrieved from https://www.nursingcenter.com/career/guideto-certification

Smith, L. (2015). Choosing a pathway: PhD or DNP? *Nursing2018,* 45(8), 20-24. doi: 10.1097/01.NURSE.0000469245.89222.6e

Chapter 11: How do I get rid of student loan debt!?!?

Seriously? ...how?

A part of this book's title is "OUTSPOKEN", therefore, I plan to be completely straightforward with the information and suggestions I provide. I only discuss what I have experienced first-hand, learned in educational programs, or learned from my peers' experiences.

How do you get rid of all your student loan debt? Honestly, I have no clue. I'm still trying to get rid of mine! The best answer I have is to budget – I guess. If your organization provides free financial counselors, use them. There are many books that discuss ways of becoming debt free.

Finances and debt are a part of my life that clearly needs some work, as with other parts. To this day, my husband leads the way with managing our finances. I am still "gaining" interest in engaging in the process of truly understanding finances – at least on a regular basis; I simply know that debt is real. Because my husband is the main "finance guy" in our relationship, I just try to be frugal in my spending.

I know. I know what you are thinking… "is she serious right now?!?!" Yes, I am. My intentions when writing this book were not to tell you how perfect I am or how successful I think I am. My goal is to let you know the truth about what exists in nursing and even in the world that surrounds or affects nursing – based on my personal experiences. All my personal experiences have not been horrible, nor have they been perfect. However, I want to be honest about what you should be doing – even though I recognize I need work in these areas as well. Many of the areas discussed in this book were from both positive and negative experiences that I have learned from and/or are continuing to learn from.

Going to school is expensive, and our economy does not allow any organization to pay you enough to *easily* live, play, take care of a family, pay off your student loans, buy a house, etc. all at the same time.

Looking back, if I could do it all over again, this is what I would have done differently as it relates to my student loans. These are thoughts I have almost every time I click the "make a payment" link and this is what you should consider.

Learned from My Experiences:

- While you may be offered a large amount of student loan money, only take/use what you need.
- If you are not financially savvy as a college or nursing student and are not sure how much student loans you need for a semester, simply take the amount offered, pay off your tuition, books, and even rent/dorm expenses (if necessary) for the entire semester. You may need to even pay an extra month of rent – if renting housing off campus to ensure you are covered and stable until your

next student loan check. After you have finished paying all required school related bills, pay close attention to how much was spent. The following semester you should feel more comfortable only getting out what you need.

- Read the details of your loan carefully!
- Pay attention to when your interest is supposed to begin accruing. If you have money after graduation, begin to pay on your student loans, even if you are in your grace period.
- Do not use your extra student loan money to go on trips or go out with friends.
- When you hear the phrase "Refund Check", remember, it is not a refund check. That phrase and the word "refund" implies that the money is yours. It is not! Not only is it not your money, the price you will have to pay for it could potentially double.
- If there is an elective at your high school (if you are still in high school) or at your college that addresses financial management, take it.
- Work a small job to pay for small bills and additional personal finances – one that does not hinder your success in the classroom.

Student loans are no joke, so do not let someone tell you differently. You may be busy studying, but if you can find time to hang out with friends and/or play intramural sports, you should be able to find time to go to your school library and check out a book that discusses how to pay back student loans. Be frugal during nursing school and plan for loan repayment prior to receiving loan repayment bills.

What I learned from Others' Experiences:

Do not overwork yourself while in nursing school (or college in general) trying to pay for school out of pocket. What do you mean Ashley? Why not just work, rather than taking out student loans?

If you do not have scholarships, grants, or other funds to pay for school and school associated financial requirements, you should work! However, pay close attention to how much you are working! If you work fulltime or too many hours, you may find yourself struggling to keep up with your school assignments.

Imagine struggling through school because you are working so much to pay for school. This will often result in either increased stress, poor grades or both. Either way, you may find yourself in a terrible cycle because some of those classes may have to be taken multiple times if you are not successful (meaning more money is required).

This statement is not meant to "promote" taking out of student loans. Your take away from this statement should be to maintain a careful balance with work, school, finances, and student loans. You are paying to go to school to get a good job to pay for "life". You do not want to find yourself paying to go to school to get a good job to pay for the schooling you already completed – struggling to pay for "life".

I'm a staff RN now, what about getting a 2nd job?

Prior to becoming a nurse, I have never heard of so many people who hold undergraduate and even graduate degrees that work two jobs to make ends meet. When I began working as a nurse, this appeared to be the norm – in nursing and in other healthcare professions. As a matter of fact, there are even many non-healthcare professionals that are working two jobs to make ends meet or to increase their income/savings. This option may or may not be an option for you, but if it is, it's worth considering. You may be able to teach clinicals as an adjunct nursing clinical instructor and allow that pay check (for one day a week as an instructor) to pay off some your student loans. If you choose to subsidize your income by being an instructor of any type, please be sure you actually care about students and their learning – please don't just chase the dollar.

However you choose to handle your student loans, just know that student loans will affect your life, so plan ahead. Having student loan debt is not the end of the world, but you should plan responsibly.

Chapter 12: Enjoying nursing

Defining success

Earlier in the book, you took some time to consider what success looks like to you. This is a term that you will have to redefine on an ongoing basis. The intent of redefining this frequently is not to change its definition repetitively because of what appears to be "failed" attempts in life. This definition of success should change because of your ongoing increased awareness and understanding about your life desires, necessities, opportunities for growth, and pathways towards attaining success.

When considering nursing as a career path or if you are still trying to navigate the nursing field, remember why you want or wanted to be a nurse. What struck your interest most about nursing? What makes you want to stay in nursing? Think about at least one thing you would like to change about your profession, your customer, and/or your work environment. Why is it necessary to change that "one thing"? Hold on to that. Let that push you through your hard days, and allow it to help you get dressed on the days you just don't feel like going in. Learn how to reward yourself and learn how to take care of yourself. There will be great days, and not so good days – of course. Don't let that derail your joy.

Do not allow any job to tear you down as an individual. Consider "who you are" outside of work. Is that the person you want to be? Your life is not and should not be "work". Nursing is hard. Sometimes enjoying nursing means moving forward down your desired path – which may mean leaving a current situation.

There will be some *written requirements* for growth and development in some nursing career pathways. These types of requirements may not be very flexible. However, you should never – ever – let anyone tell you that you "must" follow a career path that they followed in order to get to where you want to be. You will have to make some sacrifices as you develop as a nurse (and in any career path), but never sacrifice your happiness. I have been told (by a belittling and continuously demeaning supervisor) "You may be miserable now, but you are shooting yourself in the foot for leaving this job. You are making a bad choice." Five years after that statement (and after leaving), I have more than doubled my salary, have more time for myself and my family, experienced supportive colleagues and supportive leadership, increased my passion for nursing (because it *was* dwindling), and feel like I can better work towards my goals and desires for improving the nursing profession, healthcare environment, and care delivered to patients. I have cried in nursing – at work and at home. I have also learned that anything you really care about may make you cry, and that is okay. Get back up and keep moving.

I love nursing. I love what nursing is about. I enjoy improving healthcare systems – even when it's just small minute improvements. I know that each improvement will positively affect at least one patient, and that feels good. I love that there is an increasing awareness of the value of the nurse on every type of healthcare team. This awareness has led to every possible nursing career pathway you can imagine. I love knowing my career is limitless and has very few boundaries.

For me, success is loving what I do. Success also means that I am at a place where I have truly begun to understand why I do it. Success is when I can positively discuss the "what and why" behind my job to my children and my husband and they are proud of the positive work I do – not because they understand it in that moment, but because they see the pride I take in my work. Success is when I am able to spend quality time with my family without always thinking about work. (The reality is, you will think about work at home, period.) Success is learning how to let go of "the perfect" life and "the perfect" home but learning to appreciate the time I have with my family and to appreciate the outcomes and results of my hard work at home and at work. Success is when I've gotten to a place in life where I can be honest about "how I did it wrong" in order to help someone else. Success is the feeling I get when I receive feedback from someone I've helped, and they have had at least one of the same feelings I've had regarding my definition of "success".

That's my definition...
What's yours?

I hope this book provided some quick insight into the world, especially the career path, of nursing. These were all my personal views, perspectives, opinions, experiences and career choices. They do not reflect any level of perfection or lead to anyone's *absolute* "success story".

Thanks for allowing me to be... OUTSPOKEN.

Author's Note

OUTSPOKEN? While writing this, I often looked at the my title to make sure this was truly "fitting" for the book and for me. I wanted to be sure the title spoke to who I am and what I am about. "OUTSPOKEN" speaks to who I am. It is my *at home inner self* coming out – outside my home. It is the beginning of many OUTSPOKEN texts that allow me to be me in explaining my perspectives on different aspects of life.

I began working on this particular text when I was made aware about career day at my daughter's school. It became clear that I would have to soon start having conversations with my daughters about "what they want to be when they grow up". I quickly realized that I wanted my daughters to understand "what's really going on around them" – without taking away their childhood. My girls are currently five and two years old, and I want them to maintain their appropriate and expected levels of naivety.

So, as I began to contemplate on how I can communicate with my girls about what life planning looks like – even for a child, I also thought about my many experiences as "an adult". While reflecting on my college relationships, work relationships, mentoring relationships, relationships with my students, and even my relationships with patients, I realized that there is so much "growth" that happens during and after school. I have always been taught to speak up, ask questions, do what is right, help others, be a good person, state my opinion if I don't agree with something, not to allow people to run over me, respect everyone, be a Christian, remain "a lady" (whatever that means), etc. However, having lived just a little, I quickly recognized that doing all these at the same time is a challenge.

This challenge has often led to me having to decide where and when to "hold back". How do I hold back something that could be deemed as a positive trait or quality? This type of "holding back" was done to ensure that I kept my job, because sometimes doing what is right goes against the mission of my employer. This type of "holding back" was sometimes done to "just finish school" so I could keep my head down and maintain low stress levels, even though I knew my peer was being disrespected by my faculty – in front of me. Sometimes this meant adjusting and assimilating to a work culture that has decided that mediocre productivity is enough, because my colleagues are only at work to make money – not to work. Yes, I have done all these things. Yes, I have assimilated to environments that were not quite positive. However, I decided I was done. I was and I am done keeping my head down. Will I be abrasive about what I have to say and my opinions on matters that affect other people (patients, students, peers, etc)? No. But I am done being silent. I am done feeling like I can only have certain conversations about life, work, and home in a work break room. I'm even done feeling like I should keep information that should be "under the table", well...under the table.

When invited to "the table" at any point in life and asked for my input or opinion, I will not be biting my tongue. Should there be a delay in my response, it will only be due to my creative mental planning to ensure my honesty is still tactful.

I do not plan to expose people or organizations. But being OUTSPOKEN is my opportunity to let people coming after me know that "life" exists. I also want them to know that the feelings associated with life are very normal. When I was dealing with some of the experiences discussed in this book, I felt as though "I was the only one". Furthermore, I am the only healthcare professional in my entire family, so describing some of these experiences to others often felt like I was speaking another language. But this book mentions not only my experiences, but it also mentions some of my former colleagues' experiences. My knowledge of their experiences often derived from them trying to let me know that my own experiences and feelings are normal.

Will there be people that don't agree with everything I have to say? Yes. Will there be people that feel like it's not necessary to shed light on areas of life and/or nursing that are negative and don't happen everywhere? Yes. Unfortunately, not talking about these things means that those who experience any of this are subject to thinking their feelings are abnormal. That's not acceptable.

My entire life is not nursing, so you can expect OUTSPOKEN to be more than just nursing. This is just the first of being OUTSPOKEN.

Made in the USA
Monee, IL
04 November 2026

67378024R00056